Coffee Connoisseur
The complete guide

A coffee drinkers bible to understanding, buying and brewing the best coffee.

John Greco

Copyright © 2017 John Greco

All rights reserved.

ISBN-13: 978-1548227142

ISBN-10: 1548227145

DEDICATION

My family and friends who support me and encourage me to excel in life and always keep learning.

Acknowledgments

Special thanks to: Mike Kenneally Photo contributor

Marc Wortman @ makegoodcoffee.com

Maxwell House Coffee; Division of Kraft Foods Inc.

CoffeeAM.com Roaster and supplier of fresh coffee

CONTENTS

	Acknowledgments	i
1	Story of the Bean	Pg 9
2	The Purchase	Pg 20
3	Grind & Brew	Pg 34
4	Medical Research	Pg 39
5	Final Conclusions	Pg 44
6	Coffee Drinks	Pg 47
7	Cooking with Coffee	Pg 63
	About Author	Pg 81
	References	Pg 83

PREFACE

During a recent trip to Southern Italy it was almost impossible to find a cup of American coffee. The closet I came was a can of instant freeze dried coffee with a strange name on the label. Not sure if it would taste like what I wanted, I tried it and became frustrated as it was gross to say the least. I was going to pack 2 pounds of my coffee in my suitcase but decided not at the last minute. I was warned in advance but did not heed the warnings.

In southern Italy the only way a person can get a cup of coffee they are accustom to is the Italian version which is a weak, watered down espresso. Needless to say, it was like drinking hot water with a hint of burnt coffee flavor. For 2 weeks I had no choice but to drink the freeze dried make- believe cup of what I think may have been chicory coffee or several cups of espresso to satisfy my silly coffee craving.

After missing my American coffee for what seemed like a year, upon return to America, the first thing I did was make a full pot of my favorite blend of Kona and Jamaican Blue mountain fresh ground coffee. That first taste was like sex in the afternoon when I was young. Satisfying and so enjoyable. For me, it is normal to drink a 12 cup pot of coffee in the morning and more during lunch and after diner.

The experience of not having my morning fix and 50 years of tasting and later experimenting with different blends of coffee beans led me to think that somewhere out there must be a complete coffee drinkers guide to the best cup of coffee, right? I couldn't find one that had everything to know about understanding, selecting, grinding and brewing a commodity that is used everyday by tens of millions of people on a regular basis.

Don't get me wrong. There are plenty of books on and about coffee on the market, but none have a complete list of everything to do with the beans, types, origins, selections, processes, curing, roasting types, roasters, companies, blends, and different process of cutting, blending, grinding, and finally brewing using different processes. They were missing the desire for consumers who wanted to learn in great detail what they were drinking and how to make the experience better.

That alone persuaded me to write the complete guide to a coffee drinkers addiction and quest for the perfect cup of coffee.

CHAPTER 1
STORY OF THE BEAN

The story that an Ethiopian goat herder discovered coffee when his berry-eating goats became frisky and experienced the same effects while tasting it himself. Later years, it was crushed and poured into hot water to extract the beans flavor and oils to better carry the tasteful concoction into the fields for liquid consumption and energy.

Ethiopian people say that the birth of coffee as we know it started in their country. Coffee production in Ethiopia is a longstanding tradition. Ethiopia is where Coffea arabica, the coffee plant, originates. The plant is now grown in various parts of the world; Ethiopia itself accounts for around 3% of the global coffee market. Coffee is important to the economy of Ethiopia; around 60% of foreign income comes from coffee, with an estimated 15 million of the population relying on some aspect of coffee production for their livelihood.

Coffee ingestion on average is about a third of that of tap water in North America and Europe. Worldwide, 6.7 million metric tons of coffee were produced annually in 1998–2000, and the forecast is a rise to seven million metric tons annually by 2010.

As of the writing of this book, Brazil, is now the second largest consumer of coffee in the world.

Brazil remains the largest coffee exporting nation, however Vietnam tripled its exports between 1995 and 1999 and became a major producer of robusta seeds. Indonesia is the third-largest coffee exporter overall and the largest producer of washed arabica coffee. Organic Honduran coffee is a rapidly growing emerging commodity due to the Honduran climate and rich soil it produces an excellent coffee bean.

The two most economically important varieties of coffee plant

are the Arabica and the Robusta; 75–80% of the coffee produced worldwide is Arabica and 20% is Robusta. Arabica beans consist of 0.8–1.4% caffeine and Robusta beans consist of 1.7–4% caffeine. As coffee is one of the world's most widely consumed beverages, coffee beans are a major cash crop and an important export product. In 2006, coffee exports brought in $350 million, equivalent to 34% of that year's total exports. Increasing every year since providing some of the best coffee beans found in the world. Ethiopia is the world's seventh largest producer of coffee, and Africa's top producer, with 260,000 metric tonnes in 2006. Half of the coffee is consumed by Ethiopians, and the country leads the continent in domestic consumption. Worldwide consumption is about 145 million
bags of coffee a year - that's almost 10 million tons of coffee.

The world's 6 biggest coffee consumers
Brazil 2.8 cups
Netherland 2.4 cups
Finland – 2.1 cups
Norway – 1.9 cups
Iceland – 1.7 cups
Denmark – 1.5 cups
U.S.A. is 16th, less than 1 cup

Regional varieties
Ethiopian Sidamo beans

Ethiopian coffee beans that are grown in either the Harar, Sidamo, Yirgacheffe or Limu regions are kept apart and marketed under their regional name. These regional varieties are trademarked names with the rights owned by Ethiopia.

Genika
"Ethiopia Genika" is a type of Arabica coffee of single origin grown exclusively in the Bench Maji Zone of Ethiopia. Like most African coffees, Ethiopia Guraferda features a small and greyish bean, yet is valued for its deep, spice and wine or chocolate-like

taste and floral aroma. The most distinctive flavour notes found in all Sidamo coffees are lemon and citrus with bright crisp acidity. Sidamo coffee includes Yirgachefe Coffee and Guji Coffee. Both coffee types are very high quality.

Harar

Harar is in the Eastern highlands of Ethiopia. It is one of the oldest coffee beans still produced and is known for its distinctive fruity, wine flavor. The shells of the coffee bean are used in a tea called hasher-qahwa. The bean is medium in size with a greenish-yellowish color. It has medium acidity and full body and a distinctive mocha flavor. Harar is a dry processed coffee bean with sorting and processing done almost entirely by hand. Though processing is done by hand, the laborers are extremely knowledgeable of how each bean is categorized.

Bean varieties

Ethiopian coffee beans of the species Coffea arabica can be divided into three categories: Long-berry, Short-berry, and Mocha. Long-berry varieties consist of the largest beans and are often considered of the highest quality in both value and flavor. Short-berry varieties are smaller than the Long-berry beans but, are considered a high grade bean in Eastern Ethiopia where it originates.

Mocha variety is a highly prized commodity. Mocha Harars are known for their pea-berry beans that often have complex chocolate, spice and citrus notes.

Growing regions typically offer moderate sunshine and rain, steady temperatures around 70°F (20°C), and rich, porous soil. In return the delicate tree yields beans that are an economic mainstay for dozens of countries and about 25 million people—and, among natural commodities, have a monetary value surpassed only by oil. Of the two main coffee trees, Arabica beans are considered the better beans, and accounts for about 70 percent of the harvest. The harsher beans of the hardier robusta bean account for about 30 percent.

Top Ten Coffee-Producing Countries
produced during the 1997-98 crop year, according to the U.S. National Coffee Association

Brazil (22.5 million bags)
After arriving from French Guiana in the early 18th century, coffee quickly spread and thrived in Brazil. Today Brazil is responsible for about a third of all coffee production, making it by far the heavyweight champion of the coffee-producing world. Though many connoisseurs believe that Brazil's emphasis on quantity takes a toll on quality, many also praise the country's finer varieties. Brazil is the only high-volume producer subject to frost. The devastating 1975 frost, in particular, was a boom to other coffee-growing countries. Two 1994 frosts raised prices worldwide. Specific Beans: Bahia, Bourbon Santos

Vietnam (10.8 million bags)
French missionaries first brought coffee to Vietnam in the mid-1860s, but production remained negligible as late as 1980. In the 1990s, however, Vietnamese coffee production has been ratcheted up at a furious pace. Beans: Vietnam specializes in robusta production.

Colombia (10.5 million bags)
Colombia is the only South American country with both Atlantic and Pacific ports—an invaluable aid to shipping. The crop's economic importance is such that all cars entering Colombia are sprayed for harmful bacteria. Colombia's coffee grows in the moist, temperate foothills of the Andes, where the combination of high altitude and moist climate makes for an especially mild cup.Beans: Medellin, Supremo, Bogotá

Indonesia (6.7 million bags)
The Dutch unwittingly gave coffee a nickname in the late 17th century, when they began the first successful European coffee plantation on their island colony of Java (now part of Indonesia). Top-grade arabicas are still produced on Java as well as on Sumatra, Sulawesi, and Flores, but the Indonesian archipelago is most notable as the world's largest producer of robusta beans.
Beans: Java, Sumatra, Sulawesi (Celebes)

Mexico (5 million bags)
Coffee came to Mexico from Antilles at the end of the 18th century, but was not exported in great quantities until the 1870s. Today approximately 100,000 small farms generate most Mexican coffee, and most of the beans come from the south. Mexico is the largest source of U.S. coffee imports. Beans: Altura, Liquidambar MS, Pluma Coixtepec

Ethiopia (3.8 million bags)
The natural home of the arabica tree and the setting for most of coffee's origin legends, Ethiopia is Africa's top arabica exporter and leads the continent in domestic consumption. About 12 million Ethiopians make their living from coffee, whose name is said to be a derivation of "Kaffa," the name of an Ethiopian province.
Beans: Harrar, Sidamo, Yirgacheffe

India (3.8 million bags)
According to legend, India is the birthplace of coffee cultivation east of Arabia. Today coffee production is under the strict control of the Indian Coffee Board, which some say reduces economic incentive and thereby lowers quality. Beans: Mysore, Monsooned Malabar

Guatemala (3.5 million bags)
German immigrants initiated serious coffee cultivation in Guatemala in the 19th century. Today the country's high-grown beans, particularly those grown on the southern volcanic slopes,

are among the world's best. Beans: Atitlan, Huehuetenango

Côte d'Ivoire (3.3 million bags)

In the mid-1990s Côte d'Ivoire was the number five coffee producer and second largest robusta producer. Today most exports end up as mass-market coffee in Europe, especially France and Italy. Bean: Côte d'Ivoire specializes in robusta production.

Uganda (3 million bags)

Though Uganda grows precious little arabica, it is a key producer of robusta. That humble, hardy bean accounts for 75 percent of the country's export revenue and provides employment for 80 percent of all rural workers. Efforts to diversify aside, Uganda is likely to remain beholden to the bean for the foreseeable future.

As you notice there are various names for specific beans and the regions where they are cultivated. The short story to remember is the bean types: Long-berry, Short-berry, and Mocha, also known as a pea-berry as it is the smallest of the group. The type of the bean makes the taste desired. All beans should have a smoothness and complexity with no off-flavors. The beans should be neither under-roasted nor charred, and the brew should have at least moderate aroma and flavor, and subtle top notes. Some sourness and bitterness are desirable, too, to keep the coffee from tasting bland.

All coffee beans consist of arabica or robusta beans, or a combination. Arabica beans are more expensive and tend to make better coffee. And where the beans are grown makes a difference. Coffee is cultivated across the world in the Tropics of Cancer and Capricorn. Coffee drinkers have become more discriminating in recent years and coffee drinkers are demanding more flavor from their cup of Java. Consider How You Taste it. And hopefully the information above will help you in choosing the right bean to suit you desired results to the perfect cup of coffee. Arabica and robusta are the two main types of beans for all coffee. Robusta beans are less expensive and easier to grow. Arabica beans tend to make better coffee.

Did you know that coffee is one of the most chemically treated crops in the world?
Up to 250 pounds of chemical fertilizers are sprayed per acre of non-organic coffee.

When you sip your conventional coffee, you are ingesting the pesticide residues that leach into the bean, which contribute to many health problems including cancer and miscarriages in pregnant women.

Americans drink about 400 millions cups of coffee every day, and most of the coffee beans are imported. The U.S. Department of Agriculture has little control over the type and amount of pesticides used on imported coffee. Simply said, they cannot control other countries use or type of pestisides that are used and outlawed by United States.
The most effective way to protect against potential harm from the pesticides is to drink organic coffee. It will cost you more however, ask yourself just one question. Am I worth it?

Roasting is what turns green beans into coffee that is ready to grind and brew. The main types of roasting gives coffee beans different flavors in the end result.

Light Roast
Light roasting produces beans that are light brown and have a more sour taste.

Medium Roast
Medium roast coffees have medium brown beans. The beans do not have an oily surface in this roast. The coffee beans can have a bright acidity, but specific varietal aromatics (e.g. floral, fruity, chocolate, berry, etc.) of the coffee are still apparent.

Dark Roast
The beans in this roast have some oil on the surface and the color is rich and darker. The characteristics of the coffee are complemented by caramelized notes such as nutty, bread or baked goods, or bitter, and the acidity has faded somewhat, bringing out a

slightly bittersweet aftertaste. French roast is a good example.

Darker Roasts

The darkest roasts have shiny black beans with an oily surface. In a good/well done dark roast, there is still some good acidity to liven the cup. Dark roasts run the gamut from slightly dark to extremely dark. Italian roast and French roast are the darkest roasts. Not all beans are graded, with the only exception being the green coffee bean (un roasted). Green Coffee Beans Sizing Chart

1/64 inch	mm	Classification	Central America and Mexico	Colombia	Africa and India
20	8	Very Large	Superior	Supremo	AA
19.5	7.75	Very Large	Superior	Supremo	AA
19	7.5	Very Large	Superior	Supremo	AA
18.5	7.25	Large	Superior	Supremo	AA
18	7	Large	Superior	Excelso	A
17	6.75	Large	Superior	Excelso	A
16	6.5	Medium	Segundas	Excelso	B
15	6	Medium	Segundas	Excelso	B
14	5.5	Small	Terceras		C

Grading roasted beans

Roasted or harvested beans for roasting are only rated by the origins of the bean and every country rates them differently. There is no real standard of rating. There is however a loosely approved method of rating the quality of a harvest based on defects and infestation by insects into the bean.

Depending on the color of the roasted beans as perceived by the human eye, they will be labeled as light, medium light, medium, medium dark, dark, or very dark. A more accurate method of discerning the degree of roast involves measuring the reflected light from roasted seeds illuminated with a light source in the near-infrared spectrum. This elaborate light meter uses a process known as spectroscopy to return a number that consistently indicates the roasted coffee's relative degree of roast or flavor development.

Roast characteristics

The degree of roast has an effect upon coffee flavor and body. Darker roasts are generally bolder because they have less fiber content and a more sugary flavor. Lighter roasts have a more complex and therefore perceived stronger flavor from aromatic oils and acids otherwise destroyed by longer roasting times. Roasting does not alter the amount of caffeine in the bean, but does give less caffeine when the beans are measured by volume because the beans expand during roasting. **In fact, green beans have more caffeine than espresso beans** due to the expansion of the espresso beans and the temperatures at which they are roasted.
The lighter the bean, the more caffeine.

Decaffeinated coffee

Decaffeination may also be part of the processing that coffee seeds undergo. Seeds are decaffeinated when they are still green. Many methods can remove caffeine from coffee, but all involve either soaking the green seeds in hot water (often called the "Swiss water process") or steaming them, then using a solvent to dissolve caffeine-containing oils. Decaffeination is often done by processing companies, and the extracted caffeine is usually sold to the pharmaceutical industry or beverage companies for their use in energy drinks.

The Specialty Coffee Association Method of Coffee Grading

Keep in mind this is green bean only. There is no uniform standard for roasted beans except for a method called cupping.

Three-hundred grams of properly hulled coffee beans are sorted using screens 14, 15, 16, 17, and 18. The coffee beans remaining in each screen is weighed and the percentage is recorded. Since classifying 300 grams of coffee is very time consuming, 100 grams of coffee is typically used unless the quality is so good that more is needed, than 300 grams are used.

Specialty Grade Green Coffee (1): Specialty green coffee beans have no more than 5 full defects in 300 grams of coffee.

Premium Coffee Grade (2): Premium coffee must have no more than 8 full defects in 300 grams. Primary defects are permitted.

Exchange Coffee Grade (3): Exchange grade coffee must have no more than 9-23 full defects in 300 grams.

Below Standard Coffee Grade (4): 24-86 defects in 300 grams.

Off Grade Coffee (5): More than 86 defects in 300 grams.

With all that said, you would be hard to find this rating on the labels as most, if not all do not publish it on their labeling.

There are 2 coffee beans that stands in a class all its own. One special bean is only hand harvested and very rare as well as extremely expensive. Kopi Luwak is this special beans name. The other is Thailand's black Ivory coffee bean

In order to make the world's most expensive coffee from this specific bean, Kopi Luwak must be eaten by the Asian palm civet cat-like creature. Yes I did say eaten by this special type cat creature. The Civet only lives in Sumatra, Java and Bali. The creature will eat the cherry bean and the digestive acids in the stomach break down the chemical acids in the bean. Farmers dig through the scat dropping's and clean the bean removing all residue and clean it again several times more before roasting this perfectly balanced, chemically altered bean. It is said that partially digested bean have a shorter peptide chain and more free amino acids, which makes the taste of this coffee publicized as the best coffee money can buy.

In Thailand, black ivory coffee beans are fed to elephants whose digestive enzymes reduce the bitter taste of beans collected from dung. These beans sell for up to $1,100 a kilogram ($500 per lb), achieving the world's most expensive coffee some three times costlier than beans harvested from the dung of Asian palm civets.

One cup can cost between $20.00 and $90.00 depending where you purchase this outrageously priced cup of coffee.
I have tried it and it is quite unique in flavor. Earthy and a slight floral flavor with some minute nodes of chocolate, yet smooth and rich all rolled up in one package of flavor. Too expensive for my taste and out of reach by most coffee drinkers.

A new-comer on the market is a coffee variety called Centroamericano, part of a new class of F1 hybrid varieties, earned a score of 90 out of 100 points at the Nicaragua Cup of Excellence, the world's leading competition and award for high quality coffees.

The coffee took second place in the Nicaragua competition and was grown by Gonzalo Adán Castillo Moreno. Mr. Moreno's farm, Las Promesas de San Blas, is in the Northern region of Neuva Segovia, near the border with Honduras. Prices vary and production is limited in quantity.

CHAPTER 2
THE PURCHASE

From the latest preparation techniques to sourcing the beans themselves, the new generation of coffee lovers isn't satisfied with their parent's drip coffee.

Daily consumption of espresso-based beverages has nearly tripled since 2008, according to the latest data.
Between 2008 and 2016, past-day consumption of gourmet coffee beverages soared from 13% to 36% among 18-24 year olds, and from 19% to 41% for those 25-39.
For espresso-based beverages alone, the jump become 9% to 22% for the 18-24 group and 8% to 29% for those 25-39.
While the number of cups consumed in the U.S. may have declined slightly in 2016, the retail earnings have continued to increase. The food service coffee market alone increased 14.2% over the past 4 years, according to research from Packaged Facts.

As many marketers have realized, Millennia's, whose purchasing power is growing (with about $200 billion in purchasing power each year) are very picky about their coffee.
21% of coffee drinkers would be interested in having ready-made coffee delivered to their home or workplace and 16%would consider having freshly roasted ground coffee sent to their home, according to the research agency Mintel.

Now that you have learned about the beans and the different types of beans that are grown, the question becomes? What flavor are you looking for? Caffeine? How much caffeine? Caffeine or decaf? The choices are massive when you consider that a coffee bean from a certain region has different nodes of flavor. Light, dark, medium or espresso? Blended beans or one type of bean? Whole beans or ground? Choosing the right cup or pot of coffee can be quite confusing as you can see. Do you know what type of coffee you are drinking when you buy it in a chain stores? If you are happy with your coffee, close the book and enjoy life every day. If are interested in knowing more and wish to find that perfect

blend that satisfies you and causes you to want more throughout the day, then let me show you how to enrich your knowledge of coffee and choose that perfect blend of java.
Question 1: What kind of flavor do you really like? As I stated above, there are various flavor's in a coffee bean

- **Africa Regions** Bright and Fragrant
- **Central and South America regions** Mild and Smooth
- **Indonesia & South Pacific Regions** Full Bodied and Bold

First, you'll need to figure out if you like a light, medium or a dark roasted coffee.

Each specialty coffee requires different degrees of heat and roasting time to achieve its optimum flavor. What this means is that a Sumatran will require more heat (and need to be darker roasted) than say, a Colombian would, to get the most flavor out of it. If a coffee is under-roasted it will be bitter, but if over-roasted, some of the flavor will be roasted out, and it will taste a bit flat and slightly burnt in flavor

African coffee beans are usually acidic in flavor, and often have a dry, bright taste. Kenyan, Tanzanian and Zimbabwe are good examples of coffees with these characteristics. Ethiopian coffees from Harrar can have floral, fruity tastes, while those from Yrgacheffe are known for their chocolaty tones.

The coffees from the Americas are usually smooth, crisp and clean with bright aftertastes. Examples of these are Costa Rican, Guatemalan, Mexican and Colombian. Colombian coffees are the most consistent tasting from year to year. Some of these coffees, like those from Brazil & Nicaragua, have a nutty, or buttery smooth taste.

Hawaiian, Kona have a sweetness to it that makes it a truly special cup of coffee, which makes it more desirable and expensive for a select few coffee lovers.

Caribbean coffees like Blue mountain Jamaican have a close likeness to the Kona bean with a more earthy finishing flavor.

Indonesian coffees have good body, and bold flavor. Some call this taste "strong", but strong coffee is just extra coffee grind in the brewing process. Coffees from this region include Sumatra, Java, Sulawesi and India among others.

Choose the flavor you wish to try from the above list and start with that bean, if you find the flavor not to your liking try another.

Roasting coffee transforms the chemical and physical properties of green coffee beans into roasted coffee products. The roasting process is what produces the characteristic flavor of coffee by causing the green coffee beans to change in taste. Unroasted beans contain similar if not higher levels of acids, protein, sugars, and caffeine as those that have been roasted, but lack the taste of roasted coffee beans due to the other chemical reactions that occur during roasting.

The vast majority of coffee is roasted commercially on a large scale, but small-scale commercial roasting has grown significantly with the trend toward "single-origin" coffees served at specialty shops. Some coffee drinkers even roast coffee at home as a hobby in order to both experiment with the flavor profile of the beans and ensure the freshest possible roast.

Blended beans

Many commercial sellers resort to a blend of beans to reach a satisfying taste using mostly Arabica beans grown in different regions. Very few will use Arabica and Robusta due to the extra cost of the Robusta bean and its supply.

If you buy coffee in any place except Starbucks, chances are it is a Columbian Arabica roasted bean. Starbucks uses more Robusta beans for the strong flavor and body. They do have Arabica beans which is straight coffee, no added flavors.

Light roast coffee

Light Roast Coffee Beans are beans roasted at a lower temperature for a shorter period of time when compared to medium and dark roasts. Light roasting is typically at first crack, although there are variations of Light Roast. Light roast coffee beans don't seem to have the following that the medium and dark roasts. It is important to note that green and light roast beans are higher in acidity as well as antioxidants due to the lower temperatures of roasting.

Brands to try are:

Starbucks Veranda Blend™ Whole Bean Coffee.

Magnum Coffee Taste of the Exotics Coffee.

Cafe Don Pablo Subtle Earth Organic Gourmet Coffee – Light Roast.

Tiny Footprint Coffee Organic Whole Bean Coffee.

Our friends @ CoffeeAM.com have a great website to help decide on what flavor you are looking for in a fresh roasted and home delivered coffee, or just take their test on a flavor you may be looking for. Make sure to tell them Mr. John Greco recommended you to the site, for a discount on your order (If you order any of their fine fresh roasted coffee's).

Light roast include all green beans as they are not roasted and fall into the same category.

As the beans darken to a deep brown, the origin flavors of the bean are eclipsed by the flavors created by the roasting process itself. At darker roasts, the "roast flavor" is so dominant that it can be difficult to distinguish the origin of the beans used in the roast.

Medium roast

The most consumed type in America is Arabica bean from various regions and roasted to the specifications of the producers standards. The variety and flavors are different from producer to finished product. This could be based on the blend of beans, the amount of certain beans compared to another, the harvest itself and a host of other complex processes performed at the plant. Examples are: most major brands stay exact to the taste they are known for such as Maxwell House, which is a full body medium to slightly dark roast. The flavor is consistent and they are an American icon, thanks to advertisements from the 1950's to the 1980's.

I grew up on Maxwell house coffee until the changes started to take hold in the late 1980's to present. Thanks to new innovations in the coffee industry like Starbucks and Dunkin Donuts to name a few who saw a marketable product by making fancy cafés using various blends of beans and flavor extracts.

If you're looking for a smooth, full body, slightly floral and mildly acidic flavor, then this is your kind of coffee. Medium roast Arabica coffee is the most popular here in America, but don't expect to find this blend in southern Italy anywhere, it doesn't exist.

Dark roast

Becoming more popular with franchises like Starbucks and other coffee houses due to the added variety of flavors and blending of creamers used. It is impossible to taste the real flavor of the original coffee bean itself due to it being combined with never-ending additives of flavors like caramel and chocolates to name a few.

Full City+ Roast

This type of roast is considered dark. But, is just a step north of medium roasts.

Vienna Roast

A *Vienna* style roast is the next step up from Full City+.

With the additional time, more coffee bean oils are released making this type of roast have a somewhat caramel flavor.

French Roast

With a French roast, you are definitely noticing the darker color of the roasted beans. These beans will be almost shiny with oil as the beans have had a long time to release their inner oils.

French is often used in espresso drinks and with the extra oils can be extra good at creating a smooth flavor blende coffee

Italian Roast

Strong, often enjoyed because almost all of the acidity has been cooked out of the bean. With a temperature of 473°F, an Italian roast can almost be considered burnt.

Italian roast is also a favorite for espresso drinkers and exclusive to all regions of Italy. Something to remember is the darker the roast the less acidity and caffeine. It chemically strips them out due to the higher heating process. Green and light roast beans have much more acidity and caffeine.

Blending your own signature coffee:

Different areas of the same country can also make different bean flavors within the same soil substrate. The minerals in the soil make the difference in the taste stronger or weaker. Volcanic regions tend to produce stronger earthy bold flavors then low lying areas which hold more water and washed minerals that settle to the bottom of basins.

Note: Acidity is tricky and misunderstood. Don't think of acid as in pH content of coffee, or acid reflux (heartburn). Think of it as a piece of caramel candy and a chocolate bar, both have unique flavors, but which one has more "pop"? If you answered chocolate, it's the same concept behind acidity. How much "pop" would you like in your coffee? A lot can be too much, but not enough can be boring.

Choose a flavor that interest you from the descriptions below. Once you have chosen a flavor you would like to try, follow these 5 cardinal rules to ensure the best, freshest flavor.

If you want to bypass the various choices from below and want to get right down to it, try a traditional Columbian (Arabica) coffee which is the most common in the U.S.A. and a blend of any of the beans listed below to produce your special cup of bliss.

Rule # 1 The lighter the bean, the more the caffeine.

Rule # 2 The fresher the beans roast date, the more flavor.

Rule # 3 Buy whole bean and grind your own.

Rule # 4 Never freeze or refrigerate coffee.

Rule # 5 Store your beans in air-tight container.

List compiled by www.MakeGoodCoffee.com

Flavors to select from

South American Coffee

Brazilian

Flavor Characteristics

- **Complexity:** Simple

- **Acidity:** Low - of the most popular and accessible coffees of the world, Brazils have the lowest acidity
- **Body:** Medium
- Facts about Brazilian coffee
- **Facts:** Brazil is the world's largest coffee producer and produces approximately 25% of the world's coffee.
- **Region:** South America - largest area, easternmost
- **Main growing areas:** Main growing areas: Paraná, Espirito Santos, São Paulo, Minas Gerais, and Bahia
- **Most espresso coffees** are a very dark-roasted Brazilian coffee.

Colombian

Flavor Characteristics

- **Complexity:** Simple and balanced
- **Acidity:** High
- **Body:** Heavy
- Aroma: Floral

Facts about Colombian coffee...

- **Facts:** It is not the world's largest producer of coffee, but the best-marketed and most brand-recognized.
- **Region:** South America - northeast, connecting to Central America
- **Main growing areas:** Huila, Santander, Popayan, and Nariño

Central American Coffee

Costa Rican

Flavor Characteristics

- **Complexity:** Simple and balanced
- **Acidity:** High

- **Body:** Heavy

Facts about Costa Rican coffee

- **Facts:** The area's best coffee is identified by the Strictly Hard Bean designation.
- **Region:** Central America, south of Nicaragua, west of Panama
- **Main growing areas:** Tarrazu, Tres Rios, Herediá, and Alajuela

Guatemalan

Flavor Characteristics (see Coffee Taste Terms):

- **Complexity:** Complex - a "busy" flavor
- **Acidity:** High
- **Body:** Medium-high
- **Aroma:** Floral, spicy

Facts about Guatemalan coffee

- **Facts:** For what it's worth, Guatemalan Coffee is MakeGoodCoffee.com's favorite coffee of the world.
- **Region:** Latin America, east of Mexico, west of Honduras
- **Main growing areas:** Antigua, Fraijines, Huehuetenago
- **The expert** recognizes seven distinct kinds of Guatemalan coffee based on the climatically diverse soil, rainfall, and altitude in what is a relatively small country.
- **Antigua** is the most celebrated region cultivating coffee in Guatemala today. It is located in a valley between three volcanoes and has near-perfect conditions for growing coffee. Humidity is high and constant. The altitude is high, and annual rainfall is heavy.
- **Quality Control:** While private estates cultivate this coffee, a state-run board maintains quality and controlled use of the esteemed, Strictly Hard Bean (SHB) designation.

Jamaican Blue Mountain

Flavor Characteristics (see Coffee Taste Terms):

- **Complexity:** Complex and balanced
- **Acidity:** Medium
- **Body:** Heavy, rich flavor
- **Aroma:** Earthy & slightly floral

Facts about Jamaican coffee

Facts: **One of the most expensive coffee in the world.**

- **Region:** Caribbean island, south of Cuba, east of Dominican Republic
- **Main growing areas:** central Blue Mountains
- **Coffee from the Blue Mountains** of Jamaica is considered by many to be the best coffee in the world. It is also the most expensive coffee in the world, more-so even than Hawaiian Kona. It is so expensive in fact that many coffee sources do not offer it, knowing it is out of price range of the typical consumer.
- **From an online store,** expect to pay approximately $50 for a pound, and from a retail store, do not expect to find a 100% Blue Mountain blend. From a retail store, expect instead to find a cleverly named blend that likely has little real Blue Mountain beans in it.
- **The government of Jamaica** is so intent on protecting the good name of its coffee that the production and quality control is state-run. Feel free to dabble in any of the Blue Mountain blends made available at a reasonable price, but the day you really want to try Blue Mountain, buy 100% Blue Mountain from a reputable vendor.

African Coffee

Ethiopian

Flavor Characteristics

- **Complexity:** Complex and balanced - a "busy" flavor
  - **Acidity:** Medium
  - **Body:** Medium

Facts about Ethiopian coffee

- **Facts:** The birthplace of coffee.
- **Region:** Eastern Africa, east of Sudan, north of Kenya
  - **Main growing areas:** Yirgacheffe, Harar
- **This is where it all began.** All coffee originates from trees that grew in Ethiopia, and its beans that traded between itself and neighboring Yemen.
- **Ethiopian coffee** is still one of the most celebrated coffees in the world. Look for coffees from the Yirgacheffe area.

Kenyan

Flavor Characteristics

- **Complexity:** Complex and balanced
  - **Acidity:** High
  - **Body:** Medium

Facts about Kenyan coffee

- **Facts:** A British colony, Kenya was more a tea-drinking nation and developed coffee-growing relatively late.
- **Region:** east Africa, south of Ethiopia, north of Tanzania
- **Main growing areas:** Mt. Kenya, Aberdare, Kisii, Nyanza

Yemeni Mocha

Flavor Characteristics

- **Complexity:** Complex and balanced
  - **Acidity:** High
- **Body:** Medium-heavy
  - **Aroma:** Floral

Facts about Yemeni Mocha coffee

- **Fact:** The most popular and common coffee from this country is Yemen Mocha, one of two parts in the infamous Mocha Java blend.
  - **Region:** south of Saudi Arabia, east of Ethiopia
  - **Main growing areas:** central mountains of Yemen
- **Yemeni Mocha Coffee Name:** This coffee comes with the most general confusion in name. The Mocha in Yemeni Mocha coffee makes reference to the old port of Mocha from which this country's coffee and neighboring Ethiopia's coffee was first exported to the world. The Yemeni Mocha coffee has nothing to do with chocolate, whereas a Cafe Mocha or Mocha Coffee or Mochachino is used to describe the mixture of coffee and chocolate.
- **Over the history of coffee,** likely the first blend of beans and what is now the world's most popular blend is the Mocha Java coffee, making reference to two different beans - the Yemeni Mocha bean and the Indonesian Java bean. For many, this is the perfectly balanced blend as it combines very wide-ranging coffee flavors but captured in a balance so that they complement each other. Yemeni Mocha's contribution to this blend is of the 'stronger' flavors...by itself, it is a very bold cup of coffee.

Asian and Pacific Coffee

Hawaiian Kona

Flavor Characteristics

- **Complexity:** Simple and balanced
- **Acidity:** High
- **Body:** Medium-high
- **Aroma:** Floral & earthy (when fresh)

Facts about Hawaiian coffee

- **Facts:** Typically the second most expensive coffee in the world.
- **Region:** Pacific Ocean
- **Main growing areas:** Kona
- **Hawaiian Kona coffee** is celebrated by experts, but is also potentially overpriced. Consider that most other coffee growing parts of the world are not rich nations and as a result, export most of their best coffee for whatever global price coffee is fetching. Hawaii, on the other hand, is in the United States and not as reliant on the world's consumption of their coffee. Short supply of the coffee also contributes to its high price, and you will usually find a 10% Kona Blend is better priced for retail than a 100% Kona Blend which would be at least triple in price to other coffees.
- **Kona is a district** of the state of Hawaii on the southwest coast of the "Big Island". Kona coffees will usually be a blend of beans from different estates of this region.
- **The unique conditions of Kona** make for unique coffee growing usually reserved for highlands, and this is certainly the most world-famous coffee out of Hawaii. Every afternoon, you could almost set your watch to the regular cloud cover and drizzle of Kona that emulates the high-growing conditions of other coffee-growing regions.
- **There have been stories** in the past of other coffees packaged as Hawaii Kona, but with today's controls and a

reputable source, you shouldn't worry about getting an impostor.

Sumatran

Flavor Characteristics

- **Complexity:** Complex
  - **Acidity:** High
  - **Body:** Medium
  - **Aroma:** Earthy

Facts about Sumatran coffee

- **Region:** Indonesian island
- **Main growing areas:** Lintongnihuta, Diari
- **Sumatran coffee** is very well-regarded among connoisseurs for a bold complex flavor, a bright acidity, and a body that is not light but also not very heavy. The acquired taste is the earthy aroma that will taste 'dirty' to some, but is a welcome nuance to some coffee drinkers.
- Very hard to find in a medium roast

If you find that one has a flavor you like and another has a body you would like with flavor, you are free to blend beans for the taste you want. Add another type of bean for a different flavor, like Harrar (Ethiopian) for a fruity floral finish taste. Ethiopian beans can be strong, so add small amounts at a time to taste.

I personally blend a Kona bean with a Guatemalan bean to produce a full body, high acidity with nodes of fruity spice. I also use a Jamaican blue mountain bean blended with Kenyan beans which produces a rich flavor of earthy tones and notes of light bitter chocolate.

CHAPTER 3
GRINDING AND BREWING

Coffee beans must be ground and brewed to create a beverage. The criteria for choosing a method include flavor and economy. Almost all methods of preparing coffee require that the beans be ground and then mixed with hot water long enough to allow the flavor to emerge but not so long as to draw out bitter compounds. The liquid can be consumed after the spent grounds are removed. Brewing considerations include the fineness of grind, the way in which the water is used to extract the flavor, the ratio of coffee grounds to water (the brew ratio), additional flavorings such as sugar, milk, and spices, and the technique to be used to separate spent grounds. Ideal holding temperatures range from 85–88 °C (185–190 °F) to as high as 93 °C (199 °F) and the ideal serving temperature is 68 to 79 °C (154 to 174 °F). The recommended brew ratio for non-espresso coffee is around 55 to 60 grams of grounds per litre of water, or two level tablespoons for a 5- or 6-ounce cup.

The roasted coffee beans may be ground by a roaster, in a grocery store, or in the home. Most coffee is roasted and ground at a roastery and sold in packaged form, though roasted coffee beans can be ground at home immediately before consumption. It is also possible, though uncommon, to roast raw beans at home.

Coffee beans may be ground in several ways. A burr grinder uses revolving elements to shear the seed; a blade grinder cuts the seeds with blades moving at high speed; and a mortar and pestle crushes the seeds. For most brewing methods a burr grinder is deemed superior because the grind is more even and the grind size can be adjusted.

The type of grind is often named after the brewing method for which it is generally used. Turkish grind is the finest grind, while coffee percolator or French press are the coarsest grinds. The most common grinds are between these two extremes: a medium grind is used in most home coffee-brewing machines.

Coffee may be brewed by several methods. It may be boiled, steeped, or pressurized. Brewing coffee by boiling was the earliest method, and Turkish coffee is an example of this method. It is prepared by grinding or pounding the seeds to a fine powder, then adding it to water and bringing it to the boil for no more than an instant in a pot called a cezve or, in Greek, a bríki. This produces a strong coffee with a layer of foam on the surface and sediment (which is not meant for drinking) settling at the bottom of the cup.

Coffee percolators and automatic coffeemakers brew coffee using gravity. In an automatic coffeemaker, hot water drips onto coffee grounds that are held in a paper, plastic, or perforated metal coffee filter, allowing the water to seep through the ground coffee while extracting its oils and essences. The liquid drips through the coffee and the filter into a carafe or pot, and the spent grounds are retained in the filter.

In a percolator, boiling water is forced into a chamber above a filter by steam pressure created by boiling. The water then seeps through the grounds, and the process is repeated until terminated by removing from the heat, by an internal timer, or by a thermostat that turns off the heater when the entire pot reaches a certain temperature.

Note: Some consider this to be burning the coffee as it re-circulates the coffee back into the grind basket by means of re-boiling the water. Sometimes leaving a bitter burnt taste in the coffee. In the old days, a pinch of salt was added to reduce the burnt flavor. Not very effective as it changed the taste of the real flavors in coffee.

Coffee may be brewed by steeping in a device such as a French press (also known as a cafetière, coffee press or coffee plunger). Ground coffee and hot water are combined in a cylindrical vessel and left to brew for a few minutes. A circular filter which fits tightly in the cylinder fixed to a plunger is then pushed down from the top to force the grounds to the bottom. The filter retains the grounds at the bottom as the coffee is poured from the container.

Because the coffee grounds are in direct contact with the water, all the coffee oils remain in the liquid, making it a stronger beverage. This method of brewing leaves more sediment than in coffee made by an automatic coffee machine. Supporters of the French press method point out that the sediment issue can be minimized by using the right type of grinder: they claim that a rotary blade grinder cuts the coffee bean into a wide range of sizes, including a fine coffee dust that remains as sludge at the bottom of the cup, while a burr grinder uniformly grinds the beans into consistently-sized grinds, allowing the coffee to settle uniformly and be trapped by the press. Within the first minute of brewing 95% of the caffeine is released from the coffee bean.

The espresso method forces hot pressurized and vaporized water through ground coffee. As a result of brewing under high pressure. As a result, the espresso beverage is more concentrated (as much as 10 to 15 times the quantity of coffee to water as gravity-brewing methods can produce) and has a more complex physical and chemical concentration. A well-prepared espresso has a reddish-brown foam called crema that floats on the surface. Other pressurized water methods include the moka pot and vacuum coffee maker.

Cold brew coffee is made by steeping coarsely ground beans in cold water for several hours, then filtering them. This results in a brew lower in acidity than most hot-brewing methods.

Nutrition

Brewed coffee from typical grounds prepared with tap water contains 40 mg caffeine per 100 gram and no essential nutrients in significant content. In espresso, however, likely due to its higher amount of suspended solids, there are significant contents of magnesium, the B vitamins, niacin and riboflavin, and 21 mg of caffeine per 100 grams of grounds.

Serving

Once brewed, coffee may be served in a variety of ways. Drip-brewed, percolated, or French-pressed/cafetière coffee may be served as white coffee with a dairy product such as milk or cream, or dairy substitute, or as black coffee with no such addition. It may be sweetened with sugar or artificial sweetener. When served cold, it is called iced coffee.

Espresso-based coffee has a variety of possible presentations. In its most basic form, an espresso is served alone as a shot or short black, or with hot water added, when it is known as Caffè Americano. A long black is made by pouring a double espresso into an equal portion of water, retaining the crema, unlike Caffè Americano. Milk is added in various forms to an espresso: steamed milk makes a caffè latte, equal parts steamed milk and milk froth make a cappuccino, and a dollop of hot foamed milk on top creates a caffè macchiato. A flat white is prepared by adding steamed hot milk (micro-foam) to espresso so that the flavor is brought out and the texture is unusually velvety. It has less milk than a latte but both are varieties of coffee to which the milk can be added in such a way as to create a decorative surface pattern. Such effects are known as latte art.

Coffee can also be incorporated with alcohol to produce a variety of beverages: it is combined with whiskey in Irish coffee, and it forms the base of alcoholic coffee liqueurs such as Kahlúa and Tia Maria. Darker beers such as stout and porter give a chocolate or coffee-like taste due to roasted grains even though actual coffee beans are not added to it.

Instant coffee

A number of products are sold for the convenience of consumers who do not want to prepare their own coffee or who do not have access to coffee-making equipment. Instant coffee is dried into soluble powder or freeze-dried into granules that can be quickly dissolved in hot water. Originally invented in 1907, it rapidly gained in popularity in many countries in the post-war period, with Nescafé being the most popular product. Many consumers determined that the convenience in preparing a cup of instant coffee more than made up for a perceived inferior taste, although, since the late 1970s, instant coffee has been produced differently in such a way that is similar to the taste of freshly brewed coffee.[citation needed] Paralleling (and complementing) the rapid rise of instant coffee was the coffee vending machine invented in 1947 and widely distributed since the 1950s.

Canned coffee has been popular in Asian countries for many years, particularly in China, Japan, South Korea, and Taiwan. Vending machines typically sell varieties of flavored canned coffee, much like brewed or percolated coffee, available both hot and cold. Japanese convenience stores and groceries also have a wide availability of bottled coffee drinks, which are typically lightly sweetened and pre-blended with milk. Bottled coffee drinks are also consumed in the United States.

Liquid coffee concentrates are sometimes used in large institutional situations where coffee needs to be produced for thousands of people at the same time. It is described as having a flavor about as good as low-grade robusta coffee, and costs about 10¢ a cup to produce. The machines can process up to 500 cups an hour, or 1,000 if the water is preheated.

CHAPTER 4
MEDICAL RESEARCH

As of the writing of this book, studies have continued to find benefits of this magic bean and its properties. Listed are but a few known facts based on long studies and research.

Coffee's antioxidants may prevent some damage to brain cells and boost the effects of neurotransmitters involved in cognitive function, say experts. Preliminary studies have noted that as coffee (or tea) intake rises, incidence of glioma, a form of brain cancer, tends to drop. Some researchers speculate that compounds in the brews could activate a DNA-repairing protein in cells—possibly preventing the DNA damage that can lead to cells becoming cancerous.

Studies link frequent coffee consumption (4 cups per day or more) with a lowered risk of developing type 2 diabetes. Scientists suspect that antioxidant compounds in coffee—cholorogenic acid and quinides—may boost cells' sensitivity to insulin, which helps regulate blood sugar.

Some studies show that moderate coffee drinkers (1 to 3 cups/day) have lower rates of stroke than non-coffee-drinkers; coffee's antioxidants may help quell inflammation's damaging effects on arteries. Some researchers speculate that the compounds might boost activation of nitric oxide, a substance that widens blood vessels (lowering blood pressure).

One analysis of nine studies found that every 2-cup increase in daily coffee intake was associated with a 43 percent lower risk of liver cancer. Possible explanation: caffeine and antioxidant chlorogenic and caffeic acids in coffee might prevent liver inflammation and inhibit cancer cells.

Health Con 1. Java Jones

If you're sensitive to caffeine, it can cause irritability or anxiety in high doses (and what's "high" varies from person to person). How?

Chemically, caffeine looks a lot like adenosine, a "slow-down" brain chemical associated with sleep and relaxation of blood vessels. Caffeine binds to adenosine receptors on nerve cells, leaving no room for adenosine to get in—so nerve cell activity speeds up, blood vessels constrict—and you get a caffeine buzz (or irritable jitters).

Cholesterol Caution

Boiled or unfiltered coffee (such as that made with a French press, or Turkish-style coffee) contains higher levels of cafestol, a compound that can increase blood levels of LDL ("bad") cholesterol. Choose filtered methods instead, such as a drip coffee maker.

Health and pharmacology
Skeletal structure of a caffeine molecule

The primary psychoactive chemical in coffee is caffeine, an adenosine antagonist that is known for its stimulant effects. Coffee also contains the monoamine oxidase inhibitors carboline and harmane, which may contribute to its psychoactivity.

In a healthy liver, caffeine is mostly broken down by the hepatic microsomal enzymatic system. The excreted metabolites are mostly paraxanthines—theobromine and theophylline—and a small amount of unchanged caffeine. Therefore, the metabolism of caffeine depends on the state of this enzymatic system of the liver.

Polyphenols in coffee have been shown to affect free radicals in vitro, but there is no evidence that this effect occurs in humans. Polyphenol levels vary depending on how beans are roasted as well as for how long. As interpreted by the Linus Pauling Institute and the European Food Safety Authority, dietary polyphenols, such as those ingested by consuming coffee, have little or no direct antioxidant value following ingestion.

Health effects

Findings have been contradictory as to whether coffee has any specific health benefits, and results are similarly conflicting regarding the potentially harmful effects of coffee consumption. Furthermore, results and generalizations are complicated by differences in age, gender, health status, and serving size.

Extensive scientific research has been conducted to examine the relationship between coffee consumption and an array of medical conditions. The consensus in the medical community is that moderate regular coffee drinking in healthy individuals is either essentially benign or mildly beneficial. Researchers involved in an ongoing 22-year study by the Harvard School of Public Health stated that "Coffee may have potential health benefits, but more research needs to be done."
Mortality

In 2012, the National Institutes of Health–AARP Diet and Health Study analyzed the relationship between coffee drinking and mortality. They found that higher coffee consumption was associated with lower risk of death, and that those who drank any coffee lived longer than those who did not. However the authors noted, "whether this was a causal or associational finding cannot be determined from our data." A 2014 meta-analysis found that coffee consumption (4 cups/day) was inversely associated with all-cause mortality (a 16% lower risk), as well as cardiovascular disease mortality specifically (a 21% lower risk from drinking 3 cups/day), but not with cancer mortality. Additional meta-analysis studies corroborated these findings, showing that higher coffee consumption (2–4 cups per day) was associated with a reduced risk of death by all disease causes.

Cardiovascular disease

Coffee is no longer thought to be a risk factor for coronary heart disease. A 2012 meta-analysis concluded that people who drank moderate amounts of coffee had a lower rate of heart failure, with the biggest effect found for those who drank more than four cups a day. Moreover, in one preliminary study, habitual coffee consumption was associated with improved vascular function. Interestingly, a recent meta-analysis showed that coffee consumption was associated with a reduced risk of death in patients who have had a myocardial infarction.

Mental health

One review published in 2004 indicated a negative correlation between suicide rates and coffee consumption, but this effect has not been confirmed in larger studies.

Long-term studies of both risk and potential benefit of coffee consumption by elderly people, including assessment on symptoms of Alzheimer's disease and cognitive impairment, are not conclusive.

Some research suggests that a minority of moderate regular caffeine consumers experience some amount of clinical depression, anxiety, low vigor, or fatigue when discontinuing their caffeine use. However, the methodology of these studies has been criticized. Withdrawal effects are more common and better documented in heavy caffeine users.

Coffee caffeine may aggravate pre-existing conditions such as migraines, arrhythmias, and cause sleep disturbances. Caffeine withdrawal from chronic use causes consistent effects typical of physical dependence, including headaches, mood changes and the possibility of reduced cerebral blood flow.

Type II diabetes

In a systematic review and meta-analysis of 28 prospective observational studies, representing 1,109,272 participants, every additional cup of caffeinated and decaffeinated coffee consumed in a day was associated with a 9% (95% CI 6%, 11%) and 6% (95% CI 2%, 9%) lower risk of type 2 diabetes, respectively.

Cancer

The effects of coffee consumption on cancer risk remain unclear, with reviews and meta-analyses showing either no relationship or a slightly lower risk of cancer onset.

Risks

Instant coffee has a greater amount of acrylamide than brewed coffee. It was once thought that coffee aggravates gastro esophageal reflux disease but recent research suggests no link.

CHAPTER 5
FINAL CONCLUSIONS

I hope by now you see how complex coffee can be and you are far more knowledgeable then the average Joe when it comes to coffee, after reading this book. Just drinking coffee without knowing everything about it will be something of the past for you now.

I Guess you can say, I was addicted to American type brewed coffee. I did not know it until the recent Italy trip and I was surprised to say the least. Prior to that, I had read several books and magazines about coffee and the differences of the beans, brewing and mixing methods. That is the single reason why I decided to write this book all about coffee, from the tree to the taste testing to brewing the best cup of coffee you can buy.
A long time ago I too was naive to coffee and just drank what everyone else was drinking, never understanding the different types of flavors I could experience in something I had every day of my life, sometimes 7 cups or more a day for years.

So, now that you have learned the ultimate knowledge of coffee, I will share with you some of my personal tricks to a perfect brew.

Columbian coffee is the most popular, however not all Columbian beans are from Columbia at all. Many countries took the plant with them and started their own plantations in south America. So South American coffee beans are a broad range of beans and flavors based on various factors such as altitude, soil condition, pesticides used, curing, roasting and price. The only consistency is the type of bean. Long-berry, Short-berry, Mocha, premium or commercial grade.
Most (not all) buy the beans for the biggest profit which is what they are in the business to do. Make a profit, as much as possible. In the late 90's specialty shops started opening up to sell quality beans at a fair price simply because they enjoyed coffee and were able to share their knowledge of a premium coffee bean to coffee drinking customers. Starbucks was the most successful followed by the already established Dunkin Donuts, who at the times prior always sold good tasting coffee without all the fancy styles of the newcomer Starbucks.
Many others have popped up around the U.S on a smaller scale

knowing they would never be as big as those mentioned above, but they were catering to a select group who just wanted choice and quality for a reasonable price. Now the internet offers the same without the brick and mortar stores. So in reality, the consumer wins with more choice and competitive pricing.

I do buy most of my fresh roasted coffee on-line and find it convenient and fair priced. With that said, I also buy from local stores when I find a bargain or a bean that tickles my fancy. So here are my personal tips for you.

Buy a quality grinder. Remember, you will be using it every day and as my father use to say "Cheap can be expensive" meaning if you buy a cheap one, expect it to break. Cuisinart mill-grinder model DBM-8 is the one. I use it 3 times a day every day. Multi grind setting and holds ½ pound of beans, also easy to clean.

As far as coffee brewing machines, there are so many to choose from .I have used a slew of different types in my life-time and always went back to a top drip machine. For fathers-day my children and wife purchased me a De'Longhi Combination Espresso & Drip Coffee Machine which works very well with both regular drip coffee and espresso or cappuccino as it has a steam wand attached. It also saves counter space by having only one machine do it all.

One: Always by from sellers who move the product fast. Example, big brand stores sell more coffee than supermarkets by a 2 to 1 margin. Sam's club, Costco, B.J's all buy in bulk and set a reasonable price. The perfect example of moving the product out quickly. That does not mean that the coffee is fresh. The supplier may have had the product in a warehouse and offered a profitable price for the buyer to purchase stock. So, **<u>Look for the dates on the labels</u>**, if there is a roast date, stay within 3 weeks of purchase date. If not look for best used by date and get the uttermost date out you can find. **<u>Whole Bean only.</u>**

Two: Specialty shops (stores) sell some of the **freshest coffee on the market.** They sell quality and quantity for a slightly higher price but they are worth it as you will certainly taste the freshness in your first cup. **Ask questions at the stores**. I say this because you want to know if you are buying Arabica or Robusta beans. There is a big difference in caffeine and flavors.

Three: Internet sellers. Prices are all over the gamut when buying on-line. Be very careful with any purchase and check out the site before coughing up your credit card info. Look for sites that have a business phone number, address and reviews. How long have they been in business? Where are they located? Can you call them? All these are important, so do your homework before buying anything. **Ask if they sell samples** of their coffee and when it was roasted. Some of the sites I have used include: **Amazon, makegoodcoffee.com and coffeeAM.com** . I **do not purchase coffee from sites like** ebay, craigslist or any sites that cannot be verified or have little info on the coffee date of roast, freshness, ect. **If they're not in the coffee business don't buy it.**

Four: By now, you know what flavor of coffee suits you or you are still trying out different beans to find that one that satisfies your desire if not try this trick.

If you drink regular coffee at home and you like it, chances are it is a mild body with slightly high acidic nodes. The after-taste can be anything, due to the manufacturer of the coffee. **Try a bean from the Americas**. They are usually smooth, crisp and clean with bright aftertastes. Examples of these are: Costa Rican, Guatemalan, Mexican and Colombian. Colombian coffees are the most consistent tasting from year to year. Some of these coffees, like those from Brazil & Nicaragua, have a **nutty, or buttery smooth taste.** Happy? If not, blend them with African beans. They are usually acidic in flavor, and often have a dry, bright taste. Kenyan, Tanzanian and Zimbabwe are good examples of coffees with these characteristics. Ethiopian coffees from Harrar can have floral, fruity tastes, while those from Yrgacheffe are known for their chocolaty tones. Somewhere in that blend you should find a perfect cup for your taste.

Five: French roast and espresso lovers have the choices of any of the darker roasted beans and the flavors vary slightly depending upon the region the beans are grown. French roast is slightly lighter than an espresso roast and are lighter in flavor.

I hope the information was helpful in your understanding of and finding that perfect cup of delicious coffee.

CHAPTER 5
COLD COFFEE DRINKS

COLD COFFEE DRINKS

Iced Coffee Shake
1 pt milk
2 oz brewed coffee
3 tbsp sugar
6 ice cubes.
Mix ingredients into blender. Blend until thick and creamy

Granita Caffe
4 oz Espresso ground coffee
8 oz sugar
2 pt cold water
1 egg white
Place water and sugar in 2 qt saucepan. Heat to boiling, and boil until sugar is completely dissolved
Remove from heat, add coffee to sugar mixture, and let sit for 10-15 minutes.
Strain liquid, and let cool.
When cold, pour syrup into covered ice tray, and place in freezer until partially frozen (30-40 min.)
Beat egg white until stiff.
Place sugar mixture into bowl, mix in egg white, and return mixture to ice tray.
Freeze until firm, and smooth, beating every 30-40 minutes to break up ice crystals.
Serve in dessert dish topped with whipped cream.

Amaretto Cooler
1 c brewed Amaretto flavored coffee
1 c milk
½ tsp vanilla
1/3 tsp almond extract
1 tbsp sugar
1/8 tsp cinnamon
Mix coffee, milk, vanilla, almond, and sugar into pitcher.
Stir until well mixed.
Pour over ice into 2 twelve ounce glasses.

Coffee Smoothie
1 cup skim milk
2 tablespoons sugar (or equivalent of sugar substitute)
2 tablespoons chocolate syrup (regular or lite)
1 tablespoon instant coffee granules
7-10 ice cubes:
Blend for two to three minutes on high speed of blender

Banana Blend
1 ripe banana
1 ½ cups cold medium roast coffee
3 tbsp sugar
3 large scoops vanilla ice cream
Cut banana into small pieces, and mix with coffee and sugar in blender.
Blend at high speed until smooth and creamy.
Add ice cream, and blend on medium speed until mixture is creamy.
Pour into 12 oz glasses and serve immediately.

Caribbean Cooler
3 c lukewarm medium roast coffee
8 lemon slices (sliced thin)
8 orange slices (sliced thin)
1 pineapple slice
Place fruit slices in large mixing bowl.
Add coffee, and stir to mix up fruit juices and coffee.
Place in freezer and chill for 1 hour.
Remove from freezer, stir again, then remove fruit.
Serve over ice in tall glass.

Espresso Cooler
1 shot espresso
1 scoop French vanilla ice cream
1 c cold milk
1 oz French vanilla syrup
Whip cream
Mix espresso, milk, syrup, and ice cream in blender.
Blend on medium speed for 2 minutes.
Pour into tall milkshake glass.
Top with whipped cream and chocolate shavings.

Continental Cooler
1 ½ c cold French roast coffee
½ tsp Agnostura Bitters
½ tsp vanilla
1 ½ tbsp sugar
1 c club soda
4 orange slices
Mix coffee, bitters, vanilla and sugar in blender.
Blend on low speed 2 minutes.
Serve over ice in 10 oz glass, 2 inches from top.
Top off each glass with club soda and orange slice.

Tropicana Coffee
4 c cold strong coffee (French or espresso roast)
1 c milk
1 tsp rum flavoring
1 tbsp sugar
1 c club soda
Mix milk, rum flavoring, and sugar in pitcher.
Stir until sugar is dissolved.
Place in refrigerator and chill for 1 hour.
Pour 1 cup chilled mixture over ice in tall glass. Add coffee, leaving 2 inches of room.
Top off with club soda.

Ice Mocha Mint
¾ c cold medium roast coffee
¼ c milk
2 tbsp chocolate syrup
2 drops mint extract
Mix coffee, chocolate syrup, mint and milk in blender.
Fill blender with ice, and blend on med. High speed until foamy.
Serve in tall glass.

Mocha Frost
2 ½ c cold strong coffee (French roast or espresso roast)
5 tbsp chocolate syrup
1 pt coffee ice cream
Mix all ingredients in blender.
Blend on medium high until smooth.
Serve in tall Sunday glasses.

Cafe Mazagran
½ c cold strong coffee (Mexican or Costa Rican recommended)
1 tsp sugar
½ cup club soda
Mix coffee and syrup.
Pour over crushed ice, and add club soda.

Coffee Float
2 ½ cups strong coffee
2 teaspoons sugar
2/3 cup cream
4 scoops of coffee flavored ice cream
1 large bottle of Coke
Sweeten coffee with sugar, and chill
Mix coffee and cream
Fill 4 glasses half full
Add 1 scoop ice cream to each glass
Top each glass with your favorite cola

Hot coffee drinks

Black Forest Cafe
8 oz French Roast Coffee 4 Tbsp. Chocolate syrup
2 Tbsp. Maraschino cherry juice
¼ c. whipped cream
1 Tbsp. Chocolate chips
2 cherries
Combine coffee, chocolate syrup, & cherry juice
Pour into 2 six oz cups.
Top with whipped cream, chocolate chips, and cherry.

Café Lait
2 c. hot French Roast coffee
2 cups hot milk
Pour from separate warm pots or pitchers into warm coffee cups simultaneously.

Cafe Olla
2 c. water
¼ c coarsely ground Mexican Coffee
2 cinnamon sticks
1 Tbsp. Brown sugar
Combine water, coffee and brown sugar in saucepan, heat to boil. Reduce heat, simmer 3-5 minutes, and strain.
Serve in warm mugs, and place cinnamon stick into mug

Tropical Mocha
1 oz coconut syrup
½ oz cherry syrup
1 oz chocolate topping
1 shot espresso
steamed milk
Combine espresso with toppings into 8 oz cup. Fill with steamed
milk, and top with foam

Mexican Coffee
2 tbsp chocolate syrup
½ cup whipped cream
¼ tsp cinnamon
½ tbsp brown sugar
2 cups espresso roast coffee

Whip together chocolate syrup, whipped cream, cinnamon, sugar and nutmeg.
Add hot coffee, mix well, and pour into 4 warm coffee mugs.
Top with whipped cream, and lightly dust with cinnamon.

Normandy Coffee
espresso roast coffee
2 c apple juice
2 tbsp brown sugar
3 orange slices
2 cinnamon sticks
¼ tsp allspice
¼ tsp cloves

Combine ingredients into 2 qt sauce pan. Bring to boil, reduce heat and simmer for 10 minutes.
Strain mixture into warm coffee pot. Pour into cappuccino cups, garnish with cinnamon stick.

Jamaican Black Coffee
6 cups espresso or French roast coffee
1 thin sliced lemon
2 thin sliced oranges
1/3 cup sugar
3 tbsp rum

Place lemons, oranges, and coffee in 2 qt saucepan. Heat to just before boiling, and add rum and sugar.
Stir until sugar is dissolved, and remove from heat. Ladle into warm coffee cups, and garnish with lemon slices.

Georgia Coffee
3 c. Espresso roast or French Roast coffee
½ c. whipped cream
1 can (16 oz) peaches
1 ½ tbsp brown sugar
¼ tsp cinnamon
1/8 tsp ginger
Drain peaches, and set aside syrup.
Combine ½ the coffee and peaches in blender, and mix on medium setting for 1 minute.

Combine 1 c cold water, sugar, cinnamon, ginger, and peach syrup in 2 qt saucepan.
Bring to boil, reduce heat, simmer for 1 minute.
Add coffee and peach mixture, stir well, and ladle into 8 oz warm coffee cups.
Top with whipped cream and serve

Turkish Coffee
1 ½ c cold water
4 tsp French Roast or Italian Roast coffee (grind fine as possible)
4 tsp sugar
Heat water in 1 qt saucepan to luke warm. Add coffee and sugar, bring to boil, stiring occasionally. Pour ½ coffee mixture into espresso cups, and bring remaining coffee back to boil. Spoon off foam into cups, fill cups, but do not stir.

TURKISH COFFEE
Cafezinho
8 tbsp Costa Rican coffee (finely ground)
2 c cold water
1 tsp sugar
Put water into 1 qt saucepan and bring to boil.
Place coffee into strainer lined with cheesecloth Pour boiling water over coffee into coffee pot or hot pitcher.
Add sugar to taste

Austrian Coffee
4 tbsp Sumatran coffee
2 tsp brown sugar
20 whole cloves
4 pieces of orange peel, cut into 3 inch x ½ inch strips
pieces lemon peel, cut to 1 inch x ½ inch strips
1 qt cold water
Place orange peel, lemon peel and cloves into bottom of coffee pot.
Brew coffee into pot, allowing it to drip onto cloves, lemon, and orange pieces.
Sweeten with brown sugar to taste

Christmas Coffee
1 c medium roast coffee
1 tbsp brown sugar
1 egg yolk
½ c cream
nut meg
Combine sugar and egg yolk, beat until smooth. Heat cream in small saucepan, and slowly mix in eggs and sugar. Heat to just before boiling. Pour coffee into 2 warm cups and top with egg and cream mixture. Gently dust with nutmeg.

Macadamia Fudge Cappuccino
2 shots Espresso
1 oz chocolate fudge syrup
1 oz macadamia nut syrup
steamed milk, (whipped)
sweetened cocoa power
In 12 oz cup, combine syrups and espresso. Fill with steamed milk, top with whipped cream, and lightly
Dust with cocoa powder

Rasberry Torte Breve
1 shot Espresso
1 oz raspberry syrup
½ oz crème de cacao syrup
steamed milk in 12 oz cup, combine syrups and espresso, and fill with steamed milk.

Java Grog
Grog Mix
2 tbsp butter (softened)
1 c brown sugar
¼ tsp ground cloves
¼ tsp nutmeg
¼ tsp cinnamon
Mix all ingredients until smooth and creamy
Divide grog mix into 6 warm 8 oz coffee mix
Add hot coffee to fill each mug, stir well

Toffee Coffee
¼ c sugar
¾ c hot water
1 ½ c hot chocolate
2 c medium roast coffee
Melt sugar in hot skillet
. Stir constantly until sugar is golden brown and melted.
Remove from heat, slowly add hot water until caramel is dissolved.
Add hot chocolate and coffee.
Place back on heat and simmer to blend.
Pour into warm coffee mugs.
Top with whipped cream if desired.

After Dinner Mint
½ lb whole bean coffee
2 tbsp mint flavoring
½ c unsweetened cocoa
Blend coffee and mint in small mixing bowl
Place on baking sheet, bake at 200 degrees for 1 hour.
Grind coffee for Espresso machine
Mix ground coffee and cocoa powder.
Brew coffee according to directions of coffee brewer.
Store leftover coffee in air tight container in freezer.

Cafe Borgia
2 cups strong Italian coffee
2 cups hot chocolate
whip cream
grated orange peel (garnish)
Mix coffee and hot chocolate
Pour into mugs
Top with whipped cream and orange peel

Caribbean (8 servings)
1 coconut
2 cups milk
4 cups strong coffee
1 tablespoon sugar
Punch two holes in to coconut, pour liquid into saucepan
Bake coconut for 30 minutes at 300 F degrees
Break open coconut, remove meat, and grate.
Mix coconut meat, coconut liquid, and milk in a sauce pan
Heat over low heat until creamy.
Strain
Toast grated coconut under broiler
Mix milk mixture, coffee, and sugar
Pour into mugs, garnish with toasted coconut.

European
1 cup strong coffee
1 egg white
1/4 teaspoon vanilla extract
2 tablespoons half and half
Beat egg white until forms soft peaks
Gently add vanilla, and continue to beat to stiff peaks are formed
Place into 2 coffee mugs
Pour coffee over egg white
top with half and half

Grog
3 cups coffee
1/2 cup heavy cream
1 cup brown sugar
2 tablespoons softened butter
1/4 teaspoon ground cloves
1/4 teaspoon ground nutmeg
1/4 teaspoon cinnamon
Peel of one large orange, broken into 6 pieces
Peel of one large lemon, broken into 6 pieces
Place one piece of each peel into cups
Mix butter, sugar, cloves, nutmeg and cinnamon
Mix coffee and cream
Pour both mixtures into cups and stir

Irish Coffee
2 cups strong coffee
2 tablespoons orange juice
2 teaspoons lemon juice
whipped cream
Mix coffee, orange juice and lemon juice
Pour into Irish whiskey glass
Top with whipped cream

Spice Coffee (8 servings)
8 tablespoons coffee grounds
8 cups water
Peel of one large orange
Peel of one large lemon
30 cloves
4 teaspoons sugar
Place coffee and spices in coffeemaker's basket
Add water and brew

Mediterranean
8 cups strong coffee
1/3 cup sugar
1/4 cup chocolate syrup
1/2 teaspoon aniseed (tied in cheesecloth)
20 cloves
4 cinnamon sticks
whip cream
orange and lemon twists
Place coffee, sugar, chocolate syrup, aniseed, cloves and
cinnamon into a sauce pan
Heat to 200 F degrees over medium heat
Strain into mugs
Top with whipped cream and twists

Cafe Speciale
Ingredients: 4 teaspoons chocolate syrup
¼ tspn nutmeg
½ cup heavy cream
1 tbsp sugar
¾ tsp cinnamon
1-½ cups extra-strength hot coffee
Put 1 teaspoon chocolate syrup into each of 4 small cups. Combine cream, ¼ teaspoon cinnamon, nutmeg and sugar. Whip until well blended Stir remaining ½ teaspoon cinnamon into hot coffee. Pour coffee into cups. Stir to blend with syrup. Top with whipped cream.

Cafe con Miel
2 cups hot coffee
1/2 cup milk
4 tbsp honey
1/8 tsp cinnamon
Heat everything until warm, but not boiling.
Stir well to dissolve honey, and serve.

Mexican
2 cups water
1/4 cup coffee grounds (ground coarsely)
1 table spoon brown sugar
1 cinnamon stick
Place all ingredients into a sauce pan
Bring to a boil, reduce heat and simmer for 5 minutes
Strain into mugs

Mexican Mocha (hot) 4 servings
1 1/2 cups strong coffee
4 teaspoons chocolate syrup
3/4 teaspoon cinnamon
1/4 teaspoon nutmeg
1 tablespoon sugar
1/2 cup whipping cream
Put 1 teaspoon of chocolate syrup into each cup
Mix Whipping cream, 1/4 teaspoon of the cinnamon, nutmeg, and sugar
Whip until you have soft peaks
Place the last 1/2 teaspoon of cinnamon into coffee, and stir
Pour coffee into cups, stir to mix in chocolate syrup
Top with whipped cream mixture

Mocha
2 cups coffee
1/3 cup cocoa
2 cups milk
1/2 teaspoon vanilla extract
1/2 cup whipping cream
1/8 tsp cinnamon
Mix cocoa, sugar, coffee and milk in a sauce pan
Heat, over medium heat constantly stirring, until simmering
Remove from heat and stir in vanilla
Pour into cups, top with whipped cream and cinnamon

Café Alpine
8 oz fresh brewed medium roast coffee
2 tbsp brown sugar
1 tsp vanilla extract
1 tsp water
Split coffee and vanilla between 2 mugs.
Dissolve the sugar in 1 tsp water, and heat in a saucepan to boiling.
Mix in the larger portion of hot water, then pour into the two mugs.

Stir well and serve.

Cafe Caribe
4 tbsp ground coffee (fine)
½ tsp grated orange peel, dried
¼ tsp cinnamon
1 inch piece of vanilla bean
1/8 tsp ground cloves
Blend ingredients well. Brew by your usual method

Nog Coffee
1 cup coffee
1 egg yolk
1/2 cup cream
dash of nutmeg
Beat sugar and egg yolk together
Place cream into sauce pan, and heat over low setting
Whisk in egg mixture
Heat to 200 F degrees
Pour coffee into to cups, and top with cream mixture
garnish with nutmeg

CHAPTER 6
FOOD RECIES

Jalapeño Cheeseburgers with Bacon and Grilled Onions

Yield
Makes 8 servings

Ingredients

Spicy Ranch Sauce
1 cup mayonnaise
1 cup sour cream
1/2 cup chopped fresh cilantro
6 tablespoons fresh lime juice
4 green onions, finely chopped
2 tablespoons minced seeded jalapeño chile
1/2 teaspoon cayenne pepper
Burgers
2 pounds ground beef
1 small onion, chopped (about 1 1/4 cups)
1/4 cup chopped fresh parsley
2 tablespoons Worcestershire sauce
1 tablespoon chopped seeded jalapeño chile
1 teaspoon salt
1 teaspoon ground black pepper
1/4 teaspoon cayenne pepper
Worcestershire-Coffee Glaze
1/3 cup light corn syrup
2 tablespoons Worcestershire sauce
2 tablespoons ketchup
1 teaspoon instant coffee crystals
2 teaspoons (packed) golden brown sugar
3 tablespoons butter
16 bacon slices

Nonstick vegetable oil spray
8 hamburger buns or 3- to 4-inch square focaccia rolls, split horizontally
8 lettuce leaves
2 cups coarsely shredded sharp white cheddar cheese
Assorted additional toppings (such as tomato and grilled onion slices)

Preparation

For spicy ranch sauce:
Whisk all ingredients in medium bowl to blend. Season sauce with salt and pepper.
For burgers:
Gently mix all ingredients in large bowl. Form mixture into eight 1/2- to 3/4-inch-thick patties. Place on small baking sheet. Cover and chill at least 2 hours and up to 1 day.
For glaze:
Stir first 5 ingredients in small saucepan over medium heat until coffee is dissolved. Remove from heat. Whisk in butter. Season glaze to taste with salt and pepper.
Prepare barbecue (medium-high heat). Working in batches if necessary, cook bacon in large skillet over medium-high heat until crisp and brown. Transfer bacon to paper towels to drain.
Spray grill rack with nonstick spray. Toast buns until golden, about 2 minutes per side. Transfer buns, cut side up, to plates. Place lettuce on each bun bottom. Grill burgers 5 minutes, basting with glaze. Turn burgers, baste with glaze, and grill until cooked to desired doneness, about 5 minutes longer for medium. Press cheese atop each burger and allow cheese to melt. Place some sauce, then 1 burger on each bun bottom. Top each with 2 slices bacon and desired additional toppings. Cover with bun top. Serve with remaining sauce.

Old-fashioned Yankee Pot-Roast
Yield feeds 6

Ingredients
2.5—3 lbs. chuck roast or bottom round roast
½ cup all-purpose flour
¼ cup olive oil
2 onions quartered
2 tsp dill weed
5 cups strong coffee (medium roast) or 2 ½ cup espresso
5 cloves garlic
1 tbs salt
1 tbs black pepper
1 cup cornstarch slurry (corn starch and water mixed)
6 medium carrots cut into 2 inches pieces
5 potatoes (for mashed potatoes)
¼ cup milk
3 tbs butter

Preparation:
In large deep pot add olive oil medium heat
Cover roast with flour evenly, add to hot oil and turn heat up.
Brown meat on all sides to crisp coating. Turn heat down to medium low.
Add onions, garlic, salt, pepper, dill and coffee to pot. Enough to cover meat at least ½ way. Cover and let simmer for 2 hours.
Turn meat and cook for additional 2 hours.
While cooking roast, last hour make mashed potatoes, using milk, butter. Keep hot during remainder of process.
Add carrots to roast and cook for additional ½ hour or until carrots are crisp to tender.
Remove meat and cover to keep hot.
Drain grease from liquid, keeping only juices.
Remove onions and carrots to small bowl and drain.
Turn heat to boil liquid and add corn starch slurry to thicken gravy.
Slice pot roast 1/8 inch thick

Braised Short Ribs in Coffee & Ancho Chile Sauce

Yield
Makes 6 servings

Ingredients

4 dried ancho chiles, stemmed, seeded, and ribs discarded
2 cups boiling-hot water
1 medium onion, quartered
3 garlic cloves, coarsely chopped
2 tablespoons finely chopped canned chipotle chiles in adobo sauce
2 tablespoons pure maple syrup
1 tablespoon fresh lime juice
3 teaspoons salt
6 lb beef short ribs
1 teaspoon black pepper
1 tablespoon vegetable oil
1/2 cup strong coffee

Preparation

Preheat oven to 350°F.
Soak ancho chiles in boiling-hot water until softened, about 20 minutes, then drain in a colander set over a bowl. Taste soaking liquid: It will be a little bitter, but if unpleasantly so, discard it; otherwise, reserve for braising. Transfer ancho chiles to a blender and purée with onion, garlic, chipotles with sauce, maple syrup, lime juice, and 1 teaspoon salt.
Pat ribs dry and sprinkle with pepper and remaining 2 teaspoons salt. Heat oil in a 12-inch heavy skillet over moderately high heat until hot but not smoking, then brown ribs in 3 batches, turning occasionally, about 5 minutes per batch. Transfer as browned to a roasting pan just large enough to hold ribs in 1 layer.
Carefully add chile purée to fat remaining in skillet (use caution, since it will splatter and steam) and cook over moderately low heat, stirring frequently, 5 minutes. Add reserved chile soaking

liquid (or 1 1/2 cups water) and coffee and bring to a boil, then pour over ribs (liquid should come about halfway up sides of meat).

Cover roasting pan tightly with foil and braise ribs in middle of oven until very tender, 3 to 3 1/2 hours. Skim fat from pan juices and serve with ribs.

Coffee-Rubbed Cheeseburgers with Texas Barbecue Sauce

Yield
Makes 8

Ingredients

Coffee rub:
1 tablespoon instant freeze dried coffee
2 teaspoons (packed) golden brown sugar
2 teaspoons freshly ground black pepper
1/2 teaspoon ground coriander
1/2 teaspoon dried oregano
1/2 teaspoon fine sea salt
Burgers:
8 slices apple-wood-smoked bacon
1 pound ground chuck (preferably grass-fed)
1 pound ground sirloin (preferably grass-fed)
8 slices smoked provolone or smoked Gouda cheese (about 8 ounces)
8 potato-bread hamburger buns
Toppings:
8 slices red onion
8 slices tomato
Texas Barbecue Sauce

Preparation

For coffee rub:
Mix all ingredients in small bowl. Can be made 1 week ahead. Store airtight at room temperature.
For burgers:
Cook bacon in large skillet until crisp. Transfer to paper towels to drain. Break in half. Gently mix chuck and sirloin in large bowl. Form meat into 8 patties, each 3 1/2 to 4 inches in diameter and 1/3 to 1/2 inch thick. Using thumb, make slight indentation in center of each burger. Burgers and bacon can be prepared 8 hours ahead. Cover separately and chill.
Prepare barbecue (medium-high heat). Sprinkle 1 teaspoon coffee rub on top side of each burger. Place burgers, rub side

down, on grill rack. Grill until slightly charred, about 4 minutes; turn.

Place 2 bacon slice halves atop each burger. Cook 3 minutes. Top each with 1 cheese slice. Cover and cook until cheese melts, about 1 minute longer. Place burgers atop bottom halves of buns. Top with onion slices and tomato slices. Spoon dollop of Texas Barbecue Sauce over. Cover with bun tops and serve, passing additional sauce alongside.

Coffee Fruitcake

Yield
Makes 2 loaves
Active Time
25 min
Total Time
7 hr (includes cooling)

Ingredients

3 1/2 cups plus 2 tablespoons all-purpose flour
2 teaspoons cinnamon
1 teaspoon salt
1 teaspoon ground cloves
1 teaspoon freshly grated nutmeg
1 lb dried currants (3 1/3 cups)
1 lb raisins (3 cups)
1 cup lukewarm strong coffee
1 teaspoon baking soda
2 sticks (1 cup) unsalted butter, softened
2 cups packed light brown sugar
4 large eggs
1 cup molasses (not robust or blackstrap)
Special equipment: 2 (9- by 5- by 3-inch) loaf pans

Preparation

Put oven rack in middle position and preheat oven to 250°F. Brush loaf pans lightly with oil, then line bottom and sides with foil, pressing corners to help adhere.
Sift together flour, cinnamon, salt, cloves, and nutmeg into a large bowl.
Toss currants and raisins with 2 tablespoons flour mixture in a bowl. Stir together coffee and baking soda in a small bowl until dissolved.
Beat together with butter and sugar in a large bowl with an electric mixer at medium-high speed until light and fluffy, 5 to 7 minutes. Add eggs, 2 at a time, beating well after each addition,

and beat in molasses. Reduce speed to low, then add flour mixture and coffee mixture alternately in batches, beginning and ending with flour mixture and mixing until just smooth. Fold in dried fruit mixture.

Divide batter between loaf pans and smooth tops by gently rapping bottom of each pan against counter.

Bake until a wooden pick or skewer inserted in center of each cake comes out clean, 2 3/4 to 3 1/4 hours (cakes may sink slightly in center). Cool pans on racks 10 minutes, then loosen foil from sides of pans with knife and turn out cakes onto racks. Peel off foil and cool cakes completely, about 3 hours.

Cappuccino-Fudge Cheesecake

Yield
Makes 12 servings

Ingredients

Crust
1 9-ounce box chocolate wafer cookies
6 ounces bittersweet (not unsweetened) or semisweet chocolate, coarsely chopped
1/2 cup (packed) dark brown sugar
1/8 teaspoon ground nutmeg
7 tablespoons hot melted unsalted butter
Ganache
1 1/2 cups whipping cream
20 ounces bittersweet (not unsweetened) or semisweet chocolate, chopped
1/4 cup Kahlúa or other coffee-flavored liqueur
Filling
4 8-ounce packages cream cheese, room temperature
1 1/3 cups sugar
2 tablespoons all-purpose flour
2 tablespoons dark rum
2 tablespoons instant espresso powder or coffee crystals
2 tablespoons ground whole espresso coffee beans (medium-coarse grind)
1 tablespoon vanilla extract
2 teaspoons mild-flavored (light) molasses
4 large eggs
Topping
1 1/2 cups sour cream
1/3 cup sugar
2 teaspoons vanilla extract
Espresso coffee beans (optional)

Preparation

For crust:
Finely grind cookies, chopped chocolate, brown sugar, and nutmeg in processor. Add butter and process until crumbs begin to stick together, scraping down bowl occasionally, about 1 minute. Transfer crumbs to 10-inch-diameter spring-form pan with 3-inch-high sides. Wrap plastic wrap around fingers and press crumb mixture firmly up sides to within 1/2 inch of top edge, then over bottom of pan.

For ganache:
Bring whipping cream to simmer in large saucepan. Remove from heat; add chocolate and Kahlúa. Whisk until chocolate is melted and ganache is smooth. Pour 2 cups ganache over bottom of crust. Freeze until ganache layer is firm, about 30 minutes. Reserve remaining ganache; cover and let stand at room temperature to use later for creating lattice pattern.

For filling
Position rack in middle of oven and preheat to 350°F. Using electric mixer, beat cream cheese and sugar in large bowl until blended. Beat in flour. Stir rum, espresso powder, ground coffee, vanilla, and molasses in small bowl until instant coffee dissolves; beat into cream cheese mixture. Beat in eggs 1 at a time, occasionally scraping down sides of bowl.

Pour filling over cold ganache in crust. Place cheesecake on rimmed baking sheet. Bake until top is brown, puffed and cracked at edges, and center 2 inches moves only slightly when pan is gently shaken, about 1 hour 5 minutes. Transfer cheesecake to rack. Cool 15 minutes while preparing topping (top of cheesecake will fall slightly). Maintain oven temperature.

For topping:
Whisk sour cream, sugar, and vanilla in medium bowl to blend. Pour topping over hot cheesecake, spreading to cover filling completely. Bake until topping is set, about 10 minutes. Transfer cheesecake to rack. Refrigerate hot cheesecake on rack until cool, about 3 hours.

Run small sharp knife between crust and pan sides to loosen cake; release pan sides. Transfer cheesecake to platter. Spoon reserved ganache into pastry bag fitted with small star tip. Pipe 6 diagonal lines atop cheesecake, spacing 1 inch apart. Repeat in opposite direction, making lattice. Pipe rosettes of ganache around top edge of cake. Garnish with coffee beans, if desired. Chill until lattice is firm, at least

6 hours. (Can be made days ahead. Wrap loosely in foil, forming dome over lattice; keep chilled.)

Tiramisu

Yield
Makes 8 to 10 servings

Active Time
30 min

Total Time
7 hr

Ingredients
2 cups boiling-hot water
3 tablespoons instant-espresso powder
1/2 cup plus 1 tablespoon sugar, divided
3 tablespoons Tia Maria (coffee liqueur)
4 large egg yolks
1/3 cup dry Marsala
1 pound mascarpone (2 1/2 cups)
1 cup chilled heavy cream
36 savoiardi (crisp Italian ladyfingers; from two 7-ounce packages)
Unsweetened cocoa powder for dusting

Preparation
Stir together water, espresso powder, 1 tablespoon sugar, and Tia Maria in a shallow bowl until sugar has dissolved, then cool.

Beat egg yolks, Marsala, and remaining 1/2 cup sugar in a metal bowl set over a saucepan of barely simmering water using a whisk or handheld electric mixer until tripled in volume, 5 to 8 minutes. Remove bowl from heat. Beat in mascarpone until just combined.

Beat cream in a large bowl until it holds stiff peaks.

Fold mascarpone mixture into whipped cream gently but thoroughly.

Dipping both sides of each ladyfinger into coffee mixture, line bottom of a 13- by 9- by 3-inch baking pan with 18 ladyfingers in 3 rows, trimming edges to fit if necessary. Spread half of mascarpone filling on top. Dip remaining 18 ladyfingers in coffee and arrange over filling in pan.

Spread remaining mascarpone filling on top and dust with cocoa. Chill, covered, at least 6 hours.

Let tiramisu stand at room temperature 30 minutes before serving, then dust with more cocoa.

Jamaican coffee brownies

Yield
Makes 15

Ingredients

Nonstick vegetable oil spray
2 cups sugar
15 tablespoons (2 sticks minus 1 tablespoon) unsalted butter
3/4 cup unsweetened cocoa powder
3 tablespoons finely ground Jamaican Blue Mountain coffee beans
1/2 teaspoon salt
3 large eggs
1 1/2 teaspoons vanilla extract
1 1/4 cups all-purpose flour
3/4 cup pecan pieces
1 cup bittersweet or semisweet chocolate chips (6 ounces)
6 tablespoons freshly brewed Jamaican Blue Mountain coffee
30 thin strips crystallized ginger

Preparation

Preheat oven to 350°F. Spray 13x9x2-inch metal pan with nonstick spray. Combine sugar, butter, cocoa, ground coffee, and salt in large metal bowl. Place bowl over saucepan of simmering water and whisk until butter melts and ingredients are blended (texture will be grainy). Remove bowl from over water; cool mixture to lukewarm if necessary. Whisk in eggs and vanilla. Sift flour over and fold in. Mix in pecans.
Spread batter in prepared pan. Bake brownies until tester inserted into center comes out clean, about 25 minutes. Cool brownies in pan.
Place chocolate chips in small bowl. Bring brewed coffee to simmer in small saucepan; pour over chips and stir until melted and smooth. Let ganache stand until cool and beginning to thicken, about 1 hour; spread evenly over brownies. (Can be made 1 day ahead. Cover; let stand at room temperature.) Cut brownies into 15 squares.

Kahlua Coffee Brownie Cheesecake

Yield: 12-14 slices
Brownie Bottom
Ingredients:
10 tbsp (140g) unsalted butter, melted
1 cup (207g) sugar
1 tsp vanilla extract
2 eggs
3/4 cup (98g) all-purpose flour
6 tbsp (43g) natural unsweetened cocoa
1/4 tsp baking powder
1/4 tsp salt
Kahlua Coffee Cheesecake

24 ounces (678g) cream cheese, room temperature
1 cup (207g) sugar
3 tbsp (24g) all-purpose flour
1 cup (230g) sour cream, room temperature
2 tbsp instant coffee granules
2 tbsp (30ml) Kahlua, warm
2 tsp vanilla extract
3 large eggs, room temperature
Chocolate Ganache

8 oz (227g) semi-sweet chocolate chips
5 tbsp (75ml) Kahlua
5 tbsp (75ml) heavy whipping cream
Kahlua Whipped Cream

1/2 cup (120ml) heavy whipping cream
2 tbsp (30ml) Kahlua
6 tbsp (43g) powdered sugar
Directions:
TO MAKE THE BROWNIE:

Preheat oven to 350°F (176°C). Line a 9-inch (23cm) springform pan with parchment paper in the bottom and grease the sides. Combine the butter, sugar and vanilla extract in a medium sized

bowl.
Add the eggs and mix until well combined.
In another medium sized bowl, combine the flour, cocoa, baking powder and salt.
Add the dry ingredients to the egg mixture and mix until well combined.
Pour the batter into the prepared pan and spread evenly.
Bake for 20-25 minutes, or until a toothpick comes out with a few moist crumbs.

To make the cheesecake filling:

In a large bowl, beat the cream cheese, sugar and flour on low speed until well completely combined and smooth. Be sure to use low speed to reduce the amount of air added to the batter, which can cause cracks. Scrape down the sides of the bowl.
Add the sour cream and mix on low speed until well combined.
In a small bowl, combine the Kahlua and coffee granules and stir until the granules are dissolved.
Add Kahlua mixture and vanilla extract to the cream cheese mixture and mix on low speed until well combined.
Add the eggs one at a time, mixing slowly to combine after each addition. Scrape down the sides of the bowl as needed to make sure everything is well combined.
6. When the brownie is done baking, reduce the oven temperature to 300°F (148°C). Remove the brownie from the oven and pour the cheesecake batter evenly over the brownie.
Wrap the outside of the pan with aluminum foil, then place the spring form pan inside another larger pan. Fill the outside pan with enough warm water to go about halfway up the sides of the spring-form pan. The water should not go above the top edge of the aluminum foil on the spring-form pan.
Bake for 1 hour 15 minutes. The center should be set, but still jiggly.
Turn off the oven and leave the door closed for 30 minutes. The cheesecake will continue to cook, but slowly begin to cool as well.
Crack the door of the oven for 30 minutes to allow the cheesecake to continue to cool slowly. This process helps prevent cracking.

Remove the cheesecake from the oven and water bath wrapping and refrigerate until firm, 5-6 hours or overnight.

To finish off the cheesecake:
To make the ganache, place the chocolate chips in a small heat proof bowl.
Combine the heavy whipping cream and Kahlua in a glass measuring cup heat just until it begins to bowl.
Pour the hot liquid over the chocolate chips and allow to sit for 2-3 minutes, then whisk until smooth.
Pour the chocolate ganache onto the top of the cheesecake and spread evenly.
To make the whipped cream, add the heavy whipping cream, Kahlua and powdered sugar to a large mixer bowl. Whip on high speed until stiff peaks form.
Pipe the whipped cream onto the top of the cheesecake.
Sprinkle the top of the cheesecake with cocoa powder, if desired.
Refrigerate until ready to serve. Cheesecake is best for 3-5 days.

Candied Espresso Walnuts

Yield
Makes about 4 cups

Ingredients

Nonstick vegetable oil spray
2/3 cup sugar
2 tablespoons finely ground espresso coffee beans
1 tablespoon instant espresso powder
1/2 teaspoon ground cinnamon
1/4 teaspoon coarse kosher salt
1 large egg white
4 cups walnut halves (about 12 ounces)

Preparation

Preheat oven to 325°F. Spray large rimmed baking sheet with nonstick spray. Whisk sugar and next 4 ingredients in small bowl. Whisk egg white in large bowl until frothy. Add walnuts; toss to coat. Sprinkle walnuts with espresso mixture and toss to coat. Spread coated walnuts on prepared sheet in single layer.
Bake 5 minutes. Slide spatula under walnuts to loosen from baking sheet and stir, rearranging in single layer. Bake until walnuts are dry to touch, about 5 minutes longer. Loosen walnuts from sheet again; cool on sheet. Candied walnuts can be made 2 weeks ahead. Store in airtight container at room temperature.

ABOUT THE AUTHOR

Born in Brooklyn, New York moved to Long Island in 1967. Moved to Orlando, Florida 1989 to work for Walt Disney World as electrical engineer, stayed with them 17 years and left to start my own business in the food industry. After some health issues I took early retirement and went back to photography doing various jobs for reputable clients in the modeling industry as well as the food industry.
Started writing novels in 2011 and have authored several books available world-wide with several more in the writing and planning process.

God and the Gods
https://www.amazon.com/God-Gods-John-Greco

Family Secrets
https://www.amazon.com/Family-Secrets-Deathbed-Confessions-Boss/

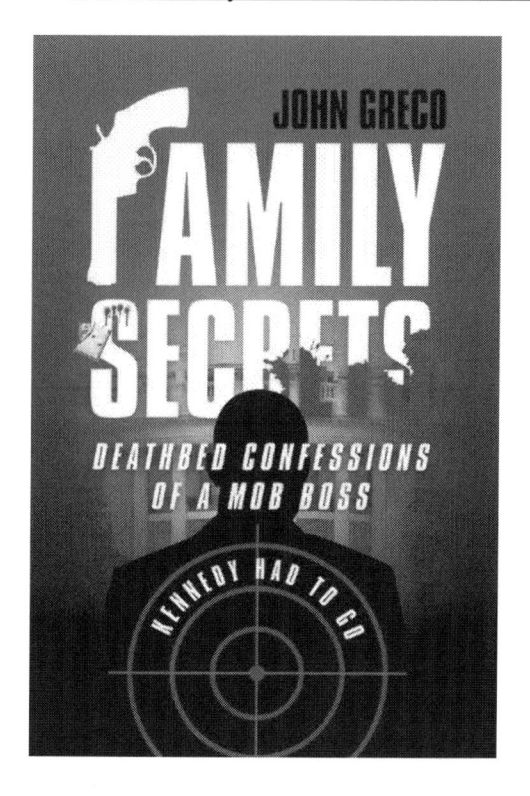

Can be reached @ https://www.facebook.com/godandthegods/
https://www.facebook.com/groups/604295339698103/
jgreco1954@outlook.com

References:

coffeescience.org/

wikipedia.org/wiki/Coffee

mnn.com/food/beverages/stories/how-coffee-changed-the-world

Made in the USA
Columbia, SC
16 January 2024